# Celebrity Diet Secrets

## Extreme Diets of the Stars

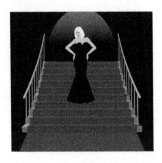

Paige Anders

Copyright © 2011 A&A publishing

**ISBN-13:**
**978-1470065867**

**ISBN-10:**
**147006586X**

# DEDICATION

To all my friends and family who have struggled with weight issues.
I hope this books let's you see that celebrities are just like us. Pot bellies and all!

*Our bodies are our gardens – our wills are our gardeners.*
*– William Shakespeare*

# Contents

Dedication
Acknowledgements
Introduction

The Raw Food Diet...................................................17

A Real Model's Diet...............................................28

Lose 5 Pounds in a week Diet.............................32

The Cigarette Diet.................................................33

The 3 Day Diet.......................................................36

The Master Cleanse Diet.......................................38

The Cabbage Soup Diet.........................................51

The Drinking Man's Diet........................................55

The Red Bull Diet...................................................58

The Apple Cider Vinegar Diet...............................60

The Grapefruit Diet...............................................64

The Cookie Diet.....................................................68

The Baby Food Diet...............................................72

# Contents

A Victoria's Secret Models Diet............................74

The Sip and Starve Diet.......................................78

What Stars are on What Diets?...........................82

About the Author.................................................96

# ACKNOWLEDGMENTS

Thanks to my editor Gary Sellers who as always, has done a great job!
All the writers that blogged into my site to leave their wonderful
recipes!
Thanks also to Health and Diet nutritional center
And also
Veronica Myers my wonderful research assistant

# Introduction

Let's face it: when it comes to celebrity diet secrets there isn't anything most of us wouldn't do get a taste of the same weight loss success that most celebrities have.

If you are looking at a few celebrity diet secrets, and wondering if they are a good option for you, it may be best to take a look at the specific regimens a certain celebrity is using.

There are many celebrity diet secrets out there that do promote effective weight loss, you just need to make sure that these methods of getting fit are actually healthy.

When you see photos of Cameron Diaz's slim silhouette or Jessica Alba's flat post pregnancy tummy you probably wonder just how Hollywood stars stay so lean or snap back into shape so quickly. While many swear their svelte bods come from eating right and exercising round the clock, the truth is that some celebs may go to strange and interesting lengths to get or stay pin thin. Here, the skinny on exactly what the big names do to get red-carpet ready—from the healthy strategies you'll want to steal to the just plain wacky ideas you'll want to avoid.

When watching E! and flipping through gossip magazines, it's hard not to wonder how stars manage to look so good. OK, maybe it has something to do with a personal trainer and that it is technically part of their job to stay in shape, but it could also be due to some of the ridiculous and slightly bizarre diets that find their way into Hollywood kitchens.

Stars like Kim Kardashian, Jennifer Aniston, and Sarah Michelle Gellar have turned to these supposed miracle weight-loss diets to help thin themselves out. So we decided to roundup some of the trendy and popular diets that have hit Hollywood and see what they're all about. Though we haven't tried any ourselves, let us know if you have (and if they work!).

## The bizarre diet secrets of the stars

It's hard to find much body fat in Hollywood.
Today's stars are slim and toned, whittled to within an inch of their lives.
When pressed about their slimming secrets, celebrities often rave about their "good genes", their affection for junk food, or declare that their secret to staying thin is simply running around after their children.
But here's what you should know: a lot of them are lying.

## Shaping up:

Angelina Jolie worked with Gunnar Peterson, who has dished the dirt on how stars achieve their figures
Celebrity trainer Gunnar Peterson, who has trained Angelina Jolie, Jennifer Lopez, and Penelope Cruz, says: "I had one actress training with me four times a week in addition to daily exercise bike classes.
When the Press asked how she'd 'transformed' her body, she said: 'Oh, I do yoga and hike with my dog.' It makes me laugh."
So the next time you see a pin-thin celebrity bragging about her relaxed approach to eating, remember this:

# They take drugs:

When Lindsay Lohan was arrested on suspicion of drink-driving, police said they found cocaine in her pocket. Paris Hilton recently admitted to U.S. talk show host Larry King that she takes Adderall for attention deficit disorder. Both drugs are often used by women looking to lose weight. Hollywood's party girls always seem to have access to certain drugs known to help shed pounds.

At the moment, Adderall is the latest diet drug craze in Hollywood, and the number of celebrities addicted to it continues to rise.

Just about every female celebrity arrested - from Paris to Nicole, from Lindsay to Britney Spears - has had prescription Adderall in her handbag. It keeps you awake while killing the appetite.

For the jet-set, hard-partying girl it has become the miracle pill - one, however, with potentially dangerous consequences. Even when taken as instructed, Adderall can cause psychotic episodes, depression and serious heart problems.

Eating disorder expert Carolyn Costin, who has treated many Hollywood actresses, says she's even seen a rise in "the drugs used for attention deficit being crumpled up and snorted". Some celebrities also take Clenbuterol, known as "Clen". Commonly prescribed to treat respiratory problems in horses, in humans it can cause fat loss.

While Clenbuterol and Adderall create a slimming effect in the short-term, after a while, users report a sudden and uncontrollable weight gain. Having tampered with the natural metabolism, the drugs stop working.

Manhattan-based trainer Justin Gelband, who works with catwalk and catalogue models, says: "Diet pills and steroids are huge right now. After Kate Moss was caught supposedly doing coke, the modeling agencies started to crack down on girls using hardcore drugs like cocaine and heroin to stay slim.

"So now it's more diet pills and steroids; they are easier to hide and, if pressed, the girls can say that they have a prescription."

They eat nothing but boiled eggs During the filming of Cold Mountain, there were rumors that one famous actress on set ate only boiled eggs.

She would rise in the morning and eat one and then have one or two at the end of the day. That was her entire diet.
And apparently she is not alone.

Celebrity trainer David Kirsch says: "I had a client who was getting ready for the Oscars and all she ate was one meal a day - of two boiled eggs! I was able to persuade her to add some almonds and a protein shake and some vitamin supplements.

"It's a self-defeating strategy, you need to eat enough, and particularly protein, to build lean and toned muscle in the first place."

**They fast:**

Paris Hilton caused a stir when she walked into New York restaurant Nobu recently.
When a waiter asked the heiress for her order, he was quietly told: "Mineral water."

In fact, over the course of her two-hour "meal", Paris took sips of water and Red Bull - she didn't eat a single bite. And she's not alone. Super-slim Desperate Housewives star Marcia Cross was spotted dining at a restaurant a few years back with her now husband Tom Mahoney.

Lifelong battle: Marcia Cross describes not eating is 'a constant struggle'

According to one eyewitness: "He ordered sea bass and prawns, but she just sipped fruit juice."
Marcia recently admitted to the pressure to be thin: "Not eating is a constant struggle. It's like they pay me not to eat. It's a living hell."

Then there's the master cleanse, otherwise known as the lemonade diet: water mixed with maple syrup, lemon juice and cayenne pepper.

Beyonce admitted following it for two weeks to drop one-and-a-half stone for the film Dreamgirls, and Jared Leto used it to shed the two stone he'd gained to play Mark Chapman in the film Chapter 27.

Gunnar Peterson calls it the "You're an idiot" diet.
"I had a client who did it and I thought he was ill," says Peterson.

"His skin was grey and his eyes had terrible dark circles under them. He was shuffling when he walked, and this was after only ten days!"

One of Hollywood's dirty little secrets is the "IV diet", in which celebrities check themselves into hospital to get put on an IV so they can avoid eating altogether.

Peterson says of the IV diet: "This is beyond ridiculous. If you're doing this you're not fat, you're crazy!"

Suzanne Peck is the director of programs at Homefield Grange Retreat, a cleansing spa in the UK that relies on juice-fasting.

She says: "Fasting is designed to rest the digestion, hence allowing clarity of thought, cleansing of toxins and healing of the body in general; not to fit into a size-zero dress."
They abuse laxative teas

Britney Spears has never been shy about her love for junk food and engages in all kinds of behaviour to counteract her taste for Taco Bell.

She smokes, drinks coffee and Red Bull, has diet pills in her bag and takes Adderall. She has also been seen hitting all-night drugstores, shopping for laxatives.
And she is certainly not alone.

Today, many actresses are taking laxatives in the form of "dieter's tea", which has a mild laxative effect. Some starlets are drinking up to ten cups a day.

Trainer Gelband says: "The latest trend among models is mixing laxative tea with the master cleanse diet. All they drink is master cleanse and laxative tea."

Such a drag: Katharine Heigl smokes regularly, a well known way of suppressing appetite

They chain-smoke Grey's Anatomy star Katherine Heigl looks to have lost a lot of weight in the last year.

She may be following a healthy eating plan, but she appears to have a secret weapon - she smokes constantly.
A few days ago, the beautiful blonde was spotted having lunch in Los Angeles. She ordered just a salad, but spent the meal chain-smoking.

Nowadays she is rarely photographed without a cigarette in her mouth, and when she isn't smoking, she is clutching a pack.

Marc David, nutritional psychologist and author of The Slow Down Diet says: "It's a choice, really. You are choosing possible lung cancer and death over treating your body with respect, all in an effort to be slim."

They eat peanuts Supermodel trainer Gelband admits: "I had one girl who was living on Diet Coke and peanuts. She drank three to five Diet Cokes a day and ate a big bag of nuts. If she got hungry, she smoked.

Her eyes had huge bags under them and she looked wasted. When we tried to work out, we had to stop every five minutes. It was awful."

**They guzzle caffeine:**

Paparazzi shots regularly show Hollywood's skinniest actresses, such as Renee Zellweger and Mary-Kate Olsen, sporting giant sunglasses and regularly coming out of Starbucks clutching gigantic cups of coffee.
This is a trend in Hollywood, where many believe coffee not only speeds up their metabolism but also keeps them from eating.

"One client I had would eat almost nothing all day, she just drank coffee constantly," says trainer to the stars Peterson. "She'd have some lettuce in the afternoon, and drink coffee instead of dinner. Working out was a waste of time because of the state she was in."

Marc David says: "Coffee and caffeine can actually make you fat. If you're drinking too much, the caffeine mimics the stress response in our bodies and your cortisol and insulin levels rise. These elevated levels of stress hormone signal the body to store fat."

**They wear a patch:**

Peterson says: "I had one guy using a Nicorette patch, not to quit smoking but to stop food cravings! This is a ridiculous approach and definitely won't work."

Gym bunny: To prepare for her role as Daisy Duke, Jessica Simpson worked out for two hours a day, six days a week

They live at the gym Who can forget those photographs of a skeletal-looking Teri Hatcher jogging through Hollywood with weights in both hands and bones protruding-through her skin?

Actress Kate Hudson, in a quest to shed the five stone she gained while pregnant with son Ryder, admitted to working out up to three hours daily for three months.

To prepare for her role as the sexy Daisy Duke, Jessica Simpson worked out for two hours a day, six days a week. Justin Gelband says: "You can get addicted. Unless you're a professional athlete, you don't need to do more than one-and-a-half hours a day to get a great result."

15

Amber Kenain, general manager at Crunch gym in Hollywood, a celeb favourite, told Glamour magazine: "There's one singer-actress who works out at my gym for about five hours a day, even on weekends. She spent her birthday here."

Peterson admits: "To be fair, a lot of the top women are doing the right things: eating healthy and exercising, but not obsessively. It's the up-and-comers who I see going to crazy extremes."

He adds: "Forget trying to look like a celebrity - look at you. The reality is, the girl that's ten pounds overweight but loves her body is winning against the girl who is underweight but hates herself.

"There's no straight guy in the world who knows the difference between a size 14 and a size 4."

# 1

## The Raw Food Diet

# Guidelines

### Green-Leafy Vegetables, Fruits, and Fats:

A fruit is any natural food containing seeds (e.g. tomato is a fruit, cucumber is a fruit). Eat fruits with seeds (avoid seedless hybrid fruit).

All types of vegetables are great, however, preference should be given to green-leafed vegetables. Avoid hybrid vegetables (i.e. carrots, beets, potatoes).

All types of raw plant foods which contain fats help transition over from cooked foods to The Raw-Food Diet. They fill you up and satiate your hunger. These include avocados, olives, coconuts, nuts, seeds, etc.

If one is sensitive to sugar, it is a good idea to add oils (flax, olive, etc.) to smoothies or fruit salads. This will allow a slower time-release of sugar into the blood. If one is extremely sensitive to sweet fruits, replace sweet fruits in the morning with grapefruits, cucumber, tomatoes, or other low-sugar fruits. Some sweet fruit, however, is necessary in the diet.

Eat nuts and seeds moderately. Quantities should be kept to less than 2.0-2.5 pounds (0.9-1.2 kg) of nuts per week. Eat nuts with green-leafed vegetables for ideal digestion. If one is sensitive to nuts, then replace all nuts listed in the menu below with avocados or olives.

All daily menus should contain a healthy balance of green-leafed vegetables (i.e. chard, collards, lettuces, kale, spinach, etc.), sugary fruits (oranges, melons, mangos, papayas, etc.), and fatty foods (i.e. avocados, olives, nuts, seeds, etc.). Chlorophyll foods build the structure of the body. Sweet fruits fuel the system with glucose. Fats lubricate and oil the body.

**Salad Dressings:** For salad dressings combine a raw plant fat with a sugar. For example, we can blend half an avocado with an orange in the blender and pour that on our salad as dressing. If we look at most commercial salad dressings on the market, we can see they consist of two basic ingredients a fat (oil, pasteurized dairy milk) and a sugar (high fructose corn syrup). People love fats and sugars with greens because they complete the Sunfood Triangle!

**Water:** The amount of water one drinks should be dictated by thirst. Raw fruits and vegetables contain so much high-quality water one may find that thirst disappears. If you drink water, drink distilled water with a squeeze of lemon at least 30 minutes before you eat a meal -- drinking water after a meal dilutes the digestive juices and interferes with digestion. If distilled water is not available, look for Evian water in glass or, if not available, in plastic.

**Alcohol:** If one drinks, s/he should preferentially choose wine over all other alcohols. Most wines have not been heat-processed. Seek out organic/no-sulfite varieties.

All beers are brewed (cooked). One should choose dark beers

with more minerals preferentially over refined commercial beers. Dark beers have a less dramatic effect on blood sugar levels.

Gradually letting go of alcohol will increase the strength of one's immune system and decrease the risk of an early death in an accident.

**Dairy Products:** Any pasteurized dairy products have long-range destructive effects on health and the digestive system. The only reason pasteurized dairy products are found in stores is because they have a longer shelf life than raw dairy products and thus they bring more money to the dairy industry.

If dairy products are included in the diet, they should be raw. Children who simply refuse to eat healthy portions of green-leafed vegetables may have raw dairy products in their diet for calcium.

Soy milk is also a bettter option than cooked milk. It has a high-fat content, and may be used to "cut" tea or coffee.

**Chewing:** Be sure to fully chew every mouthful of food. The famous Dr. Fletcher recommended 50 chews per mouthful.

Try eating with chopsticks instead of kitchen utensils as they will help to slow the rate of your eating.

## Transitional Strategy

Eat as high a percentage of raw-plant foods in your diet as possible. Feel free to eat large quantities of raw plant foods if you feel so inclined. Discover sources for raw organic foods either locally or through mail order (reference the Resources section at the end of this book). Items which may be unfamiliar such as flax seed oil or spirulina may be found at the health-food store or through mail order.

Any cooked foods should preferentially be eaten in the evening and then only one type at a time. Always combine any cooked food with the evening's large salad and freshly-made vegetable juice.

Cooked starches should be those which are lower on the Glycemic Index Chart shown in Lesson 11: The Secret Revealed, Sugar such as yams or sweet potatoes.

Transitioning off of red meat initially, then pork, chicken, and finally fish is an excellent way to let go of animal foods. For all the reasons I have outlined in this book, it is very important for our own health and success to let go of these food quickly.

Remember the simple rule: Simplicity is bliss.

Be flexible. Be easy on yourself. Transition at your own pace.

Unless otherwise stated, all menu items should be raw, plant-based, and organic.

## Quantities On The All-Raw Diet:

Feel free to eat large quantities of fruits and vegetables. You may eat less than I recommend here, however, I want you to feel free to enjoy abundant natural foods. Follow the guidelines laid out in The Sunfood Triangle. Natural raw nutrition coupled with daily exercise is the foundation of perfect health. The All-Raw Menu is designed for an active 145-175 pound (66-80 kg) individual. Those of a lighter weight and/or who are less active can adjust the quantities down accordingly.

Women, suggested daily maximum intake: 6 pounds (2.7 kg) of fruit 2.5 pounds (1.1 kg) of vegetables 0.25 pounds (0.11 kg) of nuts or seeds

Men, suggested daily maximum intake: 7.5 pounds (3.6 kg) of fruit 3 pounds (1.4 kg) of vegetables daily 0.33 pounds (0.15 kg) of nuts or seeds

# The All-Raw Diet Weekly Menu (Spring/Summer):

**Day 1:** Monday Morning: 3 pounds (1.4 kg) of watermelon (not seedless).

Afternoon: 2 mangos. 1 avocado. 3 sticks of celery.

Snack: 2 mangos.

Evening: One large lettuce, cucumber, tomato, and green onion salad with one handful of raw sunflower seeds, two avocados, and a fresh-squeezed lemon.

**Day 2:** Tuesday Morning: One large honeydew melon. The water of 2 coconuts.

Afternoon: 4 oranges. One small green-leafed vegetable salad (containing at least 3 ribs of celery) with 10-20 walnuts and fresh-squeezed lemon.

Snack: 2 oranges.

Evening: Large salad containing 80% green-leafed vegetables, 2 avocados, and an orange squeezed as dressing. 1 quart (1 liter) of freshly made vegetable juice containing at least 60% green vegetables, 40% other vegetables or fruits (i.e. apple, cucumber, yam, etc.).

**Day 3:** Wednesday Morning: 2-3 apples. 10-20 pecans or macadamia nuts with lettuce.

Afternoon: Cucumber, tomato, zucchini mixed salad. Squeeze an orange into the salad as dressing.

Snack: 2 apples. Assorted greens (green cabbage, lettuce, endive).

Evening: Large salad containing 80% green-leafed vegetables including kale or spinach eaten with 20-30 macadamia nuts, and an orange squeezed as dressing.

**Day 4:** Thursday Morning: 1/2 quart (1/2 liter) of freshly-made grapefruit juice.

Afternoon: 2 bowls of berries (strawberries, blueberries, etc.). One small lettuce salad with cucumber. 1 avocado.

Snack: 2 mangos.

Evening: Large salad containing 80% green-leafed vegetables, 20-30 almonds, and an orange squeezed as dressing. Add several servings of raw dulse seaweed to the salad.

**Day 5:** Friday Morning: 3-4 oranges (eat the white pith too!). 10-20 macadamia nuts with lettuce.

Afternoon: Cucumber, tomato, okra, zucchini mixed salad. Add high-quality extra virgin cold-pressed olive oil as dressing.

Snack: 2 oranges. Assorted greens (spinach, baby bok choy, endive).

Evening: Large salad containing 80% green-leafed vegetables, 2 avocados, and an orange squeezed as dressing. 1 quart (1 liter) of freshly made vegetable juice containing at least 60% green vegetables, 40% other vegetables or fruits (i.e. pear, zucchini, asparagus, etc.).

**Day 6:** Saturday Morning: 30-40 berries (strawberry, blueberry, etc.) mixed with lettuce or mixed with 1 avocado.

Afternoon: 1 cantaloupe. 1 quart (1 liter) of freshly made vegetable juice containing at least 50% green vegetables, 50% apples or pears.

Snack: 1 handful of sunflower seeds.

Evening: Large salad containing 80% green-leafed vegetables including 3 ribs of celery, 2 avocados, and high-quality extra virgin cold-pressed olive oil as dressing. Add several servings of raw dulse seaweed and grated raw garlic to the salad.

**Day 7:** Sunday Morning: No breakfast.

Afternoon: The water of 2 coconuts. 1 quart (1 liter) of freshly made vegetable juice containing at least 60% green vegetables, 40% other vegetables or fruits (i.e. asian pear, broccoli, cauliflower, etc.).

Snack: 2 apples. 2 ribs of celery.

Evening: Large salad containing 80% green-leafed vegetables, 1 avocado, dulse seaweed, and an orange blended with raw, unhulled tahini as dressing.

# The All-Raw Diet Weekly Menu (Fall/Winter):

**Day 1:** Monday Morning: 2 young coconuts, with coconut meat and water blended together in a cream. If young coconuts cannot be found, blend 2 avocados with mature coconut water.

Afternoon: 5 oranges. 2 avocados. Spinach leaves.

Snack: 3 oranges.

Evening: One large spinach salad containing cucumber, tomato, and green onion salad with 1 avocado and fresh-squeezed lemon.

**Day 2:** Tuesday Morning: One large papaya eaten whole or blended with orange or lime juice.

Afternoon: 4 oranges. One small green-leafed vegetable salad (containing kale or spinach) with 10-20 almonds and fresh-squeezed lemon.

Snack: 2 oranges.

Evening: Large salad containing 80% green-leafed vegetables, 2 avocados, cayenne pepper, and an orange squeezed as dressing. 1 quart (1 liter) of freshly made vegetable juice containing at least 60% green vegetables, 40% other vegetables or fruits (i.e. squash, peppers, okra, etc.).

**Day 3:** Wednesday Morning: 1 quart (1 liter) of freshly-made orange juice mixed with 1/2 avocado or 3 teaspoons of flax seed oil. (Mixing a fat with a sugar for breakfast will time-release the sugar for more endurance energy).

Afternoon: Cucumber, 10 pitted dates, lettuce mixed salad. Squeeze an orange into the salad as dressing.

Snack: 2 persimmons. Assorted green leaves (lettuce, spinach, endive).

Evening: Large salad containing 80% green-leafed vegetables eaten with 1-2 cups of raw nuts, and an orange squeezed as dressing. Add several servings of raw dulse seaweed to the salad. Add 30-40 Sun-ripened olives (if available).

**Day 4:** Thursday Morning: 2 large pomegranates and 3 oranges cut and juiced on a citrus juicer. Blend with 0.5 ounces (0.015 liters) flax oil if desired.

Afternoon: 8 dried prunes. Silicon salad! (see Appendix C: Sunfood Recipes).

Snack: 2 asian pears. Assorted greens (kale, spinach, baby

bok choy).

Evening: Nori rolls! Be creative! (see Appendix C: Sunfood Recipes).

**Day 5:** Friday Morning: 8 tangerines. 1 avocado.

Afternoon: Cucumber, okra, zucchini, onion mixed salad. Add high-quality extra virgin cold-pressed olive oil as dressing

Snack: 2 tangerines. 1 grapefruit.

Evening: Large salad containing 80% green-leafed vegetables, 2 avocados, and an orange squeezed as dressing. 1 quart (1 liter) of freshly made vegetable juice containing at least 60% green vegetables (including 3 ribs of celery), 40% other vegetables or fruits (i.e. asparagus, apple, cucumber, etc.).

**Day 6:** Saturday Morning: 1 Papaya mixed with lettuce or mixed with 1 avocado.

Afternoon: 1 cup (0.25 liters) of wheatgrass juice blended or juiced with 3-4 apples or 1 quart (1 liter) of freshly-made vegetable juice containing at least 50% celery, 50% apples or pears.

Snack: 2 apples. 10 almonds.

Evening: Large salad containing 80% green-leafed vegetables (including kale or spinach), 2 avocados, and high-quality extra virgin cold-pressed olive oil as dressing. Add 8 pitted dates to the salad for added zest.

**Day 7:** Sunday Morning: No breakfast.

Afternoon: 1 quart (1 liter) of freshly made vegetable juice containing at least 60% green vegetables (including 3 ribs of celery), 40% other vegetables or fruits (i.e. jicama, pumpkin, etc.).

Snack: 2 pears. 1 zucchini.

Evening: Large salad containing 80% green-leafed vegetables, 3 avocados, and a lemon or lime squeezed as dressing.

# 2

## A Real Model's Diet: Nyree

We thought we'd ask a top model to share her diet over a 3 day period. Here is Nyree's food diary, from 3 days earlier this year.

The best way to lose weight is to combine diet and exercise, and Nyree exercised on two of these days. Day 1 - Day 2 - Day 3

Nyree's Diet: Day 1

9:00am Breakfast
Boiled Egg with slice of wholewheat bread (140 calories)
Bowl of Cheerios with skimmed milk (220 calories)
Black Coffee (9 calories)
Total 369 calories

1:00pm Lunch
Subway Club Sandwich (320 calories)
Diet Coke (0 calories)
Total 320 calories

4:00pm Snack
Granola Bar (110 calories)

Total 110 calories

7:00pm Dinner
Grilled Chicken and steamed vegetables (360 calories)
Glass of Wine (110 calories)
Total 380 calories

9:00pm Snack
Bowl of chopped watermelon (50 calories)
Total 50 calories

Day 1 Total = 1307 calories

Nyree's Diet: Day 2

8:45am Breakfast
1 grapefruit (64 calories)
1 slice wholewheat toast, thinly spread with peanut butter
(145 calories)
Black Coffee (9 calories)
Total 218 calories

12:30pm Lunch
Turkey salad with balsamic vinaigrette (300 calories)
Cup of tea with skimmed milk (20 calories)
Total 320 calories

4:10pm Snack
Cup of apple sauce (105 calories)
Glass of orange juice (150 calories)
Total 255 calories

8:00pm Dinner
Lean Cuisine chicken a l'orange with rice (268 calories)

2 slices of low fat cheddar cheese with wholewheat crackers
(180 calories)
Total 448 calories

9:00pm Snack
Chewy granola bar (130 calories)
Total 130 calories

Day 2 Total = 1371 calories

Nyree's Diet: Day 3

9:30am Breakfast
Dannon low calorie yoghurt (90 calories)
Omelette - 2 eggs, low-fat cheese, vegetables (325 calories)
Black Coffee (9 calories)
Total 424 calories

1:30pm Lunch
Low fat BLT sandwich on wholewheat (275 calories)
Diet Coke (0 calories)
Total 275 calories

5:00pm Snack
Strawberry & Mint Salad
Total 180 calories

8:00pm Dinner
Grilled Sea Bass with vegetables (300 calories)
Glass of wine (110 calories)
Total 410 calories

Day 3 Total = 1289 calories

And there you have it, Nyree's eating habits for three full days. Remember that what works for Nyree might not work for you, so its important to try all the diet plans here and keep at it!

# 3

## Lose 5 pounds in 1 week Diet

Lose 5 Lbs of Bloat

(In a Healthy way)

Jillian Michaels recipe for losing 5 pounds in 7 days

-Get 68 ounces of distilled or pure water

-add 1 tablespoon of sugar-free cranberry juice

-add 1 dandelion tea bag

-add 2 tablespoons of lemon juice

You drink the 68 oz drink everyday for 7 days

This recipe works because it helps to flush out excess water weight you have carrying around in your body

and you could lose more than 5 pounds in 7 days depending on how much excess water weight you are carrying.

# 4

## The Cigarette Diet

GETTING THIN ON THIS DIET MAY COST YOU YOUR LIFE.

BACKGROUND
--------------------------------------------------------------------------------

THE CIGARETTE DIET IS ONE THAT DATES BACK TO THE 1920S. AT THE TIME, LUCKY STRIKE CIGARETTE COMPANY WANTED TO BOOST SALES, SO THEY USED THE APPETITE CURBING NATURE OF NICOTINE TO THEIR ADVANTAGE. WITH THE AD CAMPAIGN SLOGAN "REACH FOR A LUCKY INSTEAD OF A SWEET" LUCKY ENTICED MANY PEOPLE TO SMOKE INSTEAD OF CONSUME EXTRA CALORIES.

AND THE CAMPAIGN WORKED: SALES WERE BOOSTED OVER 200 PERCENT IN THE 1920S WITH THE USE OF THAT SLOGAN. OTHER TOBACCO COMPANIES JUMPED ON THE BAND WAGON DURING THIS TIME PERIOD AND PROMOTED SMOKING AS A WEIGHT LOSS METHOD.

YET AS MORE AND MORE RESEARCH SHOWED THE DANGER OF SMOKING, THE CIGARETTE DIET'S

TIME IN THE LIMELIGHT HAS SURELY COME TO PASS. SMOKING CAUSES MANY DEADLY DISEASES AND CONDITIONS SUCH AS LUNG CANCER AND HEART DISEASE.

UNFORTUNATELY, ALTHOUGH THE DIET WAS CREATED IN THE 1920S, IT IS STILL POPULAR TODAY AMONG TOP SUPERMODELS AND THOSE NEEDING TO KEEP THEIR WEIGHT DOWN FOR THEIR PROFESSION.

PRO
--------------------------------------------------------------------------------

•DOES LEAD TO WEIGHT LOSS
•CURBS APPETITE
CON
--------------------------------------------------------------------------------

•PROMOTES THE SMOKING OF CIGARETTES
•SMOKING CAUSES LIFE THREATENING HEALTH CONDITIONS
•SMOKING CAN AFFECT YOUR HEALTH AND THE HEALTH OF THOSE EXPOSED TO THE SMOKE
•CLASSIFIED AS A FAD DIET
DIET AND NUTRITION
--------------------------------------------------------------------------------

THERE IS NO RECOMMENDED WAY OF EATING WITH THE CIGARETTE DIET. YOU SIMPLY SMOKE AND THAT WILL SUPPRESS YOUR APPETITE AND

AID IN WEIGHT LOSS. YOU CAN BASICALLY EAT
WHAT YOU WANT.
EXERCISE
--------------------------------------------------------------------------
------

NO EXERCISE IS RECOMMENDED WITH THE
CIGARETTE DIET. THE POINT OF THE DIET IS THAT
IF YOU SMOKE, YOUR APPETITE WILL BE
SUPPRESSED AND YOU WILL LOSE WEIGHT. YOUR
LUNG CAPACITY IS LIKELY TO BE VERY
COMPROMISED CONSIDERING THE ADVERSE
EFFECTS SMOKING HAS ON THE RESPIRATORY
AND CIRCULATORY SYSTEMS OF THE BODY,
MAKING EXERCISE RATHER CHALLENGING.
CONCLUSION
--------------------------------------------------------------------------
------

THERE ARE A LOT OF DANGEROUS DIETS AND DIET
PILLS ON THE MARKET BUT THE CIGARETTE DIET
MAY TOP THE LIST AS THE MOST DANGEROUS.
ENCOURAGING PEOPLE TO SMOKE IN ORDER TO
LOSE WEIGHT COULD END UP COSTING THEM
THEIR LIFE. IN THE TIME THAT CIGARETTES WERE
HEAVILY PROMOTED AS A WEIGHT LOSS TOOL,
THE HEALTH RISKS WEREN'T KNOWN. NOW THAT
PEOPLE ARE AWARE OF THE DANGERS SMOKING
CAN CAUSE, IT IS VERY IMPORTANT THAT IT NOT
BE USED AS A WEIGHT LOSS TOOL.

LOSING WEIGHT AND BECOMING HEALTHY ARE
GOOD GOALS TO HAVE. SMOKING MAY LEAD YOU
TO WEIGHT LOSS, BUT IT WILL ALSO DAMAGE
YOUR HEALTH IN THE PROCESS.

# 5

# Three Day Diet

Super Diet Must be followed exactly!!

**Day 1**
Breakfast - Half a grapefruit, One slice of toast, 2 Tbls. of Peanut Butter

Lunch - 2 slices of any type of meat (3 oz.) 1 cup of String Beans, 1 cup f beets, 1 small apple, 1 cup of vanilla ice cream

Dinner - Half a cup of Tuna, 1 slice of toast, coffee or tea

**Day 2**
Breakfast - 1 egg, 1 slice of toast, half a banana

Lunch - 2 frankfurters, 1 cup of broccoli, hals cup of carrots, half a banana, half cup of vanilla ice cream

Dinner - 1 cup of cottage cheese, 5 saltine crackers

**Day 3**
Breakfast - 5 saltine crackers, 1 slice cheddar cheese, 1 small apple

Lunch - 1 cup of tuna, 1 cup of beets, 1 cup of cauliflower, half a banana, cantaloupe, half cup of vanilla ice cream

Dinner - 1 hardboiled egg, 1 slice of toast

Diet works on chemical breakdowns and is proven.  Do not vary or substitute any of the above foods. Salt and pepper may be used, but no other seasonings. Where there is no quantity listed you may eat all you want but use common sense.

This diet is to be used for three days at a time ONLY! In three days you will lose 10 pounds.  After the 3 day diet you can go back to normal foods...Do not overdo it! After 4 days of normal eating go back to the 3 day diet.

You can lose up to 40 pounds in a month if you stick to this diet.

Drink lots of water and you are allowed diet soda with no calories in them.

# 6

## The Master Cleanse Diet

The Master Cleanse is a 10-day fast that is used for detox and weight loss purposes. It has also been called the Master Cleanser Diet after the original book that described it, the Lemonade Diet, the Maple Syrup Diet, and the Cayenne Pepper Diet after some of the ingredients used, and the Beyoncé Diet after its most famous fan.

Although the Master Cleanse is often referred to as a fast, it's not really a complete fast, in that up to 1,300 calories are consumed each day in the form of sugars from the ingredients in the beverage that Master Cleansers prepare and drink.

The Master Cleanse was originally developed in 1940 as a stomach ulcer cure by alternative health practitioner Stanley Burroughs (1903-1991). In 1976 Burroughs presented his diet in a book, The Master Cleanser, by which time he was promoting the diet not only for ulcers, but for weight loss and "every kind of disease," claiming it would lead to "the correction of all disorders." The book is a disorganized, difficult-to-decipher jumble, and in 2004 a fan of the diet, Peter Glickman, published his more comprehensible version in the book Lose Weight, Have More Energy & Be Happier in 10 Days, dubbing it the "Lemonade Diet." Glickman's book revived the diet's popularity.

Neither Burroughs nor Glickman was a physician or medical researcher. Burroughs promoted a number of alternative practices beyond the Master Cleanse, including light therapy, deep massage, and reflexology, and he was a practicing nudist and vegetarian. He was convicted of practicing medicine without a license and imprisoned, and he was convicted of second degree murder, later overturned, for his role in the death of a desperate leukemia patient, whose cancer Burroughs tried to cure with the Master Cleanse and other practices. Glickman is a software engineer cum chiropractor who has promoted the medically rejected practice of chelation.

Among the celebrities who have been reported to have used the diet are Beyonce Knowles, who lost 20 pounds in two weeks for her role in the movie Dreamgirls, and Howard Stern sidekick Robin Quivers, who was quoted in People magazine that she heard about it from magician David Blaine and used it on three occasions while reducing her weight to 145 pounds from 218 pounds. Actor Jared Leto used the Master Cleanse to lose the 60 or so pounds that he had gained for his role as John Lennon's killer Mark David Chapman. Singers Ashanti and Trina have also been connected with the diet. Moses and Jesus both reportedly underwent a pre-Burroughs 40-day version of the diet, not involving lemonade or laxatives.

**Does it Work?**

Does the diet work for weight loss? If you follow the instructions, it most certainly will work. Any fast will cause you to lose weight, because you aren't eating food. The Master Cleanse in the strict sense is not a fast because you drink a considerable amount of sugar-containing lemonade, about 650 to 1,300 calories worth per day, depending on the number of glasses you drink. Thus you will have a daily calorie deficit: Most non-overweight people need from 1,600 to 2,400 calories per day to maintain their weight (women will be on the lower end of that range). If you are overweight, you are probably consuming more than that to maintain your weight.

As an example, if you normally eat 2,150 calories, and you choose the extreme 650-calorie version of the Master Cleanse, you will have a 1,500-calorie deficit, losing three pounds of fat per week (and perhaps some water weight also). (There may be other factors that will affect this result.) Many reputable diets prescribe a two-pound per week loss, so in this sense the Master Cleanse is actually not that radical: it just substitutes lemonade for real food and adds the shock effect of constant colon cleansing.

### Is is Dangerous? Master Cleanse Dangers

Most medical authorities don't believe that a few days of fasting will harm you (and the Master Cleanse is more of a low-calorie, nutrient deficient diet than a fast). But longer periods will begin to deplete muscle, and your heart is among the muscles that will suffer — not a good thing. In addition, longer fasts can damage your kidneys and liver. Where is the safe cut-off point? We can't really say.

Less is known about the long-term effects of 10 days or more of salt-water laxative use.

### About This Detox Stuff

Most people today, deep down, are interested in the Master Cleanse primarily for its get-skinny-quick aspect, although they rarely admit it. But there is also a detox component. What about detox?

There's no evidence that our bodies contain excessive toxins of the sort Burroughs discusses, and there's no evidence that detox diets flush out anything bad in your body. Many of our organs, including the liver, kidneys, lungs, and the intestines, are very efficient filters that expel toxins. There are toxins that may be trapped in fat cells or the lungs, but this sort of diet does not help with expelling those.

We've included some quotes from Stanley Burroughs at the end of this article so you can read for yourself how naive and outdated his medical theories were.

### How to Do the Master Cleanse

In a nutshell, the Master Cleanse is this:
■The diet takes at least 10 days (up to 40 days, the period of time that Jesus fasted after his baptism, as Burroughs points out)
■The only nourishment that you take is a special lemonade concoction made from the Master Cleanse ingredients: lemon juice, maple syrup, cayenne pepper, and water, six to twelve glasses per day, each glass containing about 110 calories in sugar carbohydrates
■An herbal laxative tea is drunk at night and a quart of salt water is drunk first thing in the morning, resulting in several liquid bowel movements every day — you need to always be near a toilet when you do this diet, and you need to stock up on toilet paper
■You come off the diet by transitioning to solid food over a few days, ideally becoming a raw food vegetarian in Stanley Burroughs' version of the diet

## Buy Master Cleanse

Master Cleanse kits are available from Peter Glickman, Coombs, Neera, and Maple Valley Syrup. All ingredients for the recipes are included, except for fresh lemons, which must be sourced locally, although some Master Cleansers bend the rules and use Lakewood 100% Organic bottled pure lemon juice.

## The Master Cleanse Lemonade

The lemonade is prepared by mixing the ingredients in this free recipe:

■2 tablespoons freshly squeezed lemon juice. Burroughs recommends organic lemons, fresh, not bottled juice. Limes may be substituted. Lemon zest and pulp may be added, making sure that the lemons are organic and not artificially colored or treated with pesticides.

■2 tablespoons of maple syrup. This must be pure maple syrup, not pancake syrup. Burroughs recommends the darker Grade B, which has more color and nutrients than Grade A, which is also acceptable. He goes into aspects of maple syrup production that would be difficult for the average person to investigate, such as whether formaldehyde or plastic tubing is used (not recommended by Burroughs).

■1/10 teaspoon cayenne pepper. Burroughs insists that cayenne chili pepper be used, but permits ramping up from a lesser amount if the taste needs getting used to.

■Water. Burroughs recommends a 10-ounce glass of medium hot water, but also allows cold water to be used. Some have interpreted "10-ounce glass" to mean 8 ounces of actual water. Since Burroughs also allows plain water to be drunk during the fast in addition to the lemonade, this doesn't seem important.

An alternative to the lemonade endorsed by Burroughs substitutes 10 ounces of fresh sugarcane juice for the lemon juice and water. But few people are going to have access to fresh, organic sugar cane juice. Some people who can not stomach the maple syrup taste have substituted an equal number of calories of powdered sugarcane or organic cane sugar, available from some health food stores (one user described it as tasting like pond scum, worse than the maple syrup).

## Things to Avoid at All Costs

Burroughs strongly counsels against the use of honey in the lemonade or the consumption at any time of honey, which he describes as predigested bee vomit, popular only among "gullible health foodists."

Burroughs also cautions against taking any kind of supplements or vitamin pills or using illicit drugs. Although Glickman wisely recommends against going off any prescription medications without your doctor's approval, it's unclear what Burroughs' opinion was on this point. He reprints without comment an endorsement from a follower who relates how he quit his medications for blood pressure, nerves, and lack of energy during his fast. And Burroughs was generally against traditional medicine in general, discouraging a leukemia patient from getting a bone marrow transplant. And an alternative version of the Master Cleanse for diabetics described in the book recommends that the diabetic phase out insulin during the diet. In another context in the book Burroughs rails against "the unnatural action of drugs and antibiotics," saying they store "poisons in the body." But we're with Glickman on this one.

You shouldn't smoke or drink alcohol, coffee, tea, cola, but the good news is that your cravings for them will completely disappear, according to Burroughs. Burroughs allows the consumption of extra plain water and of mint tea.

No other food or drink should be consumed at all, say both Burroughs and Glickman.


**The Colon Blaster**

There are two preparations needed to induce colon cleansing.
■Laxative herb tea. Although Burroughs is quite specific about types and amounts of lemons and maple syrup, on the subject of laxative herb teas he simply suggests without further elaboration that you should buy any good brand offered by your health food store.
■Internal salt water bathing solution. Dissolve two teaspoons of uniodized sea salt in a quart of lukewarm water.

The laxative herb tea and the salt water are the one-two punch that will keep your colon in full-time Old Faithful mode during the diet, cleansing it clean as a whistle.

**During the Diet**

To begin the diet you need to choose the minimum number of days that you are going to attempt, steel yourself for what is to come, and follow the following daily routine.

Day 0 (the day before beginning the diet):

Purchase lemons, maple syrup, cayenne pepper, laxative herbal tea, and sea salt in sufficient quantities to last the duration of your cleanse.

Purchase a large supply of toilet paper and Tucks® brand witch hazel wipes. If you share your bathroom with others, agree on a unque emergency code phrase like "It's coming," "Dr. Livingston, I presume," or "Elvis is leaving the building" to alert other members of your household that you need them to vacate the bathroom quickly; also, consider purchasing a supply of adult diapers.

The night before beginning the diet, drink some laxative herbal tea, and retire for the evening.

Days 1 through 10 (and Beyond):
■In the morning before drinking any lemonade, drink a quart of salt water (remain near a toilet).
■During the day drink 6 to 12 glasses of the Master Cleanse lemonade concoction. The lower number of 6 glasses is recommended for those seeking weight loss. The higher number is fine for those interested mostly in detoxification.
■In the evening drink some herbal laxative tea.
■You may experience dizziness, vomiting, joint pain, and weakness. You will also be really hungry. After several days many Master Cleanse dieters report entering a state of bliss that is either the result of the continuing elimination of toxins, or else a state similar to the tranquil experience that people who are starving to death have shortly before dying.

Note: Over the years since Stanley Burroughs' death variations of the original Master Cleanse described here have developed, and attempts at clarifying ambiguous points have been made. Peter Glickman's book, as well as this popular internet based book, deal with some of these modifications to the Master Cleanse orthodoxy.

## Post Diet: Breaking the Fast

When are you through with the diet? Either when you reach the number of days that you planned, or alternately, when your tongue goes from "coated and fuzzy" to a clear pink color.

Burroughs outlines a gentle approach for coming off the diet without upsetting your digestive system excessively. Although Burroughs recommends that you become a practicing raw foodist vegetarian after the diet to avoid recontamination with toxic dead animal flesh, he does provide an alternative transition plan for omnivores.

Vegetarian Transition Process
■Days 1 and 2: Drink several 8-ounce glasses of orange juice, sipping slowly, diluting it if there is digestive distress.
■Day 3: Drink orange juice in the morning, eat raw fruit for lunch, and eat fruit or raw salad for dinner.
■Day 4: You may return to your normal diet.

Omnivore Transition Process
■Day 1: Drink several 8-ounce glasses of orange juice, sipping slowly, diluting it if there is digestive distress.
■Day 2: Drink orange juice during the morning and afternoon. For dinner prepare a homemade vegetable soup (recipe below). Mostly sip the broth, and do not eat much of the vegetables.
■Day 3: Drink orange juice in the morning, have leftover vegetable soup for lunch with 4 rye crackers (no regular crackers or bread), and eat fresh raw vegetables, salad, and

46

fruit for dinner. Do not yet eat meat, fish, eggs, bread, pastries or drink tea, coffee, or milk.

■Day 4 and beyond: You may return to your normal diet, but Burroughs recommends continuing to drink the lemonade concoction at breakfast on a permanent basis. And he really wants you to go vegetarian, if at all possible.

Master Cleanse Recipe: The Omnivore Vegetarian Soup

Ingredients:
■2 varieties of beans, 1/2 cup each (kidney beans, lentils, pinto beans, or other)
■1 medium potato, half-inch cubes
■1 stalk celery, sliced
■1 carrot, sliced
■1 small bunch turnip greens, spinach, mustard greens or other green
■1 onion, diced
■3 medium tomatoes
■1 green pepper, diced
■1 zucchini, sliced
■1/2 cup brown rice
■Other vegetables as desired
■No meat
■1 teaspoon cumin
■1 teaspoon dry oregano
■1 teaspoon curry powder
■1/8 teaspoon cayenne pepper
■1 teaspoon salt
■vegetarian soup powder or cube (optional)

Preparation:

Combine ingredients with 4 cups water, bring to a simmer, cook 20 minutes or until potatoes and beans are tender, adding water along the way if necessary.

## Protein and the Master Cleanse

The Master Cleanse provides several hundred calories of carbohydrate per day in the form of lemon and maple sugar, and Burroughs' recommended vegetarian diet excludes "toxic dead animal flesh." What about protein? In the case of protein, Burroughs says that there is no need to worry: protein is simply nitrogen, oxygen, hydrogen, and carbon. The air contains all these elements. Simple by breathing "we are able to assimilate and build the nitrogen also into our bodies as protein ... by natural bacteria action...." But just to be on the safe side, Burroughs also recommends eating nuts and seeds after the Master Cleanse.

## Master Cleanse Alternatives

There are other cleanses out there, and many dieters spend time looking into the Master Cleanse vs. water fast, Master Cleanse vs. juice fast, and Master Cleanse vs. Colonix.

## Beyond the Master Cleanse

In addition to promoting his lemonade concoction as being useful for detoxification, weight loss, and the cure of ulcers and leukemia, Burroughs also recommended it as a baby formula. Mother's milk is best, but when not available Burroughs recommended feeding babies freshly prepared coconut milk, with the lemonade concoction given between coconut milk feedings, diluted a bit if the cayenne pepper upsets the baby. When the baby is weaned, it should be fed vegetarian foods like fruit, vegetables, berries, and seeds, sweetened with maple syrup.

Burroughs also writes of his 10- to 30-day treatment for dropsy (edema), which involves going on the Master Cleanse, and then being buried in 100-pounds of coarse rock salt purchased from a feed store, followed by steam baths.

### Quotations from Stanley Burroughs

On germs, viruses and epidemics:

"In recent times it has been believed that these many diseases are contagious and that germs have spread them....

"Disease, old age, and death are the result of accumulated poisons and congestion throughout the entire body. These toxins become crystallized and hardened, settling around the joints, in the muscles, and throughout the billions of cells all through the body ... Lumps and growths are formed all over the body as storage spots for unusable and accumulated wast products ... These growths and lumps appear to us as forms of fungi....

"When we stop feeding this fungi and cleanse our system ... they dissolve or break up and pass from the body.... Germs and viruses do not and cannot cause any of our diseases ... Germs and viruses are in the body to help break down waste material and can do no harm to healthy tissues....

"Basically, all of our diseases are created by ourselves because we have never taken the time to discover the true foods meant for man's use.

"Since germs do not cause our disorders, there must be another logical reason for the triggering of an epidemic. This is a matter of simple 'vibration.' The better the physical and mental condition a person is in, the higher becomes his vibration, but as he steadily becomes clogged with more and more waste matter, his vibration goes constantly downward...."

On his imprisonment for practicing medicine without a license:

"After dedicating a goodly share of my past life in perfecting and simplifying a system of healing that is completely free from error and side effects, at a very low cost, I was forced to overcome many difficult obstacles that often threatened to stop me, but I persisted in spite of the medical and legal attacks. I was told in each case I was doing too much good, and to keep me from giving the help that solved their health problems I was sent to prison so I couldn't help anyone any more. But ... many of the guards, nurses and even doctors [in prison] came to me for help that no other system could [offer]. In prison I was not competing with their medical rackets, but on the outside I hurt their con games. If my system was made legal, the medical system would be of no further need."

# 7

## The Cabbage Soup Diet

Diet Cabbage soup recipe :

■6 large green onions (also called "spring" onions)
■2 green peppers
■1 or 2 cans of tomatoes (diced or whole)
■3 carrots
■1 container (10 oz. or so) mushrooms
■1 bunch of celery
■half a head of cabbage
■1 package spice only soup mix (In the US, Liptons is a good choice)
■1 or 2 cubes of bouillon (optional)
■1 48oz can Low Sodium V8 juice (optional)
■Season to taste with pepper, parsley, curry, garlic powder, etc. (Little to NO SALT!)

Directions:

Slice green onions, put in a pot on medium heat and start to sauté with cooking spray. Do this until the onions are whiter/clearer in color (about 4-6 minutes).

Cut green pepper stem end off, then cut pepper in half to take out the seeds and membrane. Cut the green pepper into bite size pieces and add to pot.

Take the outer leafs layers off the cabbage, cut into bite size pieces, add to pot.

Clean carrots, mushrooms, and celery, cut into bite size pieces and toss them in. Add tomatoes now, too.

If you would like a spicy soup, add a small amount of curry or cayenne pepper now.

For seasonings, you can use a spice soup packet of your choice (no noodles!) or use beef or chicken bouillon cubes. These cubes are optional, and you can add spices you like instead (make sure not to add much salt, if any at all).

Use about 12 cups of water (or 8 cups and the 48 oz of Low Sodium V8 juice), cover and put heat on low. Let soup simmer for a long time – about 2 hours or until vegetables are tender.

Remember: This diet should only be followed for 7 days at a time, with at least two weeks in between.

Day One:

Fruit: Eat all of the fruit you want (except bananas). Eat only your soup and the fruit for the first day. For drinks-unsweetened teas, cranberry juice and water.

Day Two:

Vegetables: Eat until you are stuffed will all fresh, raw or cooked vegetables of your choice. Try to eat leafy green vegetables and stay away from dry beans, peas and corn. Eat all the vegetables you want along with your soup. At dinner, reward yourself with a big baked potato with butter. Do not eat fruit today.

Day Three:

Mix Days One and Two: Eat all the soup, fruits and vegetables you want. No Baked Potato.

Day Four:

Bananas and Skim Milk: Eat as many as eight bananas and drink as many glasses of skim milk as you would like on this day, along with your soup. This day is supposed to lessen your desire for sweets.

Day Five:

Beef And Tomatoes: Ten to twenty ounces of beef and up to six fresh tomatoes. Drink at least 6 to 8 glasses of water this day to wash the uric acid from your body. Eat your soup at least once this day. You may eat broiled or baked chicken instead of beef (but absolutely no skin-on chicken). If you prefer, you can substitute broiled fish for beef on one of the beef days (but not both).

Day Six:

Beef and Vegetables: Eat to your heart's content of beef and vegetables this day. You can even have 2 or 3 steaks if you like, with leafy green vegetables. No Baked Potato. Eat your soup at least once.

Day Seven:

Brown rice, unsweetened fruit juices and vegetables:
Again stuff, stuff, stuff yourself. Be sure to eat your soup at
least once this day.

# 8

## The Drinking Man's Diet

The Drinking Man's Diet is a fad diet that was made famous by William the Conqueror around 1087. The king had gained so much weight that he was too heavy for his horse to carry.

One day in an attempt to lose weight quickly, he stopped eating food and started drinking alcohol. Thus began The Drinking Man's Diet, which has evolved through the years and is considered an extreme and unsafe fad diet.

Today's version of the diet includes drinking martini's before lunch and eating steaks for dinner. The new version is the brainchild of Robert Cameron and his pamphlet outlining the diet sold over two million copies in 1964. Cameron has lived to be 93 and is still trim from following this diet over the years.

Overall the Drinking Man's Diet includes lowering carbohydrate consumption and encourages consumption of things certain kinds of alcohol and meat.

PRO
-----------------------------------------------------------------------
-----------

•Great for those who enjoy a good steak and a glass or two of alcohol

•Doesn't involve counting calories
•Cookbook available
•Drinking modest amounts of certain kinds of alcohol has been linked to health benefits
CON

---

•Diet restricts carbs
•May encourage binge drinking
•May promote using alcohol to control weight
•Consuming large amounts of red meat can lead to higher cholesterol levels
•Classified as a fad diet
•Those who have specific known risk factors for breast cancer should abstain from alcohol
•Not that much different from other low-carb, high protein diets
DIET and NUTRITION

---

The Drinking Man's Diet focuses on drinking alcohol and lowering carbohydrate intake. The diet originally started with just drinking alcohol and not eating at all when William the Conqueror used it in 1087. But today, it has been altered to include real food in the form of animal protein.

A sample day on the Drinking Man's Diet might look like this:

•

Breakfast: A few slices of cantaloupe, two slices of bacon, two poached or scrambled eggs, coffee or tea.

•

Lunch: Two glasses of dry wine, or one dry martini or whiskey and soda, broiled fish or steak or roast chicken, green beans or asparagus, lettuce and tomato salad with French or Roquefort dressing, and coffee or tea.

•

Dinner: Martinis or high balls, shrimp cocktail, steak, pork, lamb or chicken, one cup of low starch vegetables, 1/2 an avocado with French dressing, small serving of cheese, coffee or tea.

There are no calorie counts for the Drinking Man's Diet, but daily carbohydrate grams should be kept to 30 or fewer.
EXERCISE
-----------------------------------------------------------------------
----------

There is no formal exercise plan given.
CONCLUSION
-----------------------------------------------------------------------
----------

The Drinking Man's Diet is a low-carb diet plan with the addition of allowing a glass or two of alcohol during lunch and dinner.

While this diet is not seriously flawed, its low-carb approach might be difficult to maintain in the long-term and its allowance of alcohol a few times a day is not a recommended practice, particularly for those who have a genetic predisposition to breast cancer and to addiction.

If you have any pre-existing health conditions, do get clearance from your doctor first before following this plan.

# 9

## The Red Bull Diet

Are you overweight?

Do you want to lose 100 pounds in 8 months?

Do you enjoy drinking 10 to 14 cans of Red Bull a day?

Do you thrive on up to 1120mg of caffeine daily?

Then the Red Bull Diet is for you. According to a news story out of New Zealand an Auckland woman did just that! She claims that she would only eat at times a hand full of cereal a day along with her 14 cans of Red Bull. She started drinking this gradually and began noticing the appetite suppressing qualities of the drink so soon she was drinking up to 14 cans daily.

When Brooke Robertson, 23 years old, of New Zealand, chugged a couple Red Bulls one day, she made an unusual discovery: She wasn't hungry. This discovery snapped into place in the context of Brooke's depression about weighing 231 pounds.

For the next 8 months, Brooke ingested nothing but 10 to 14 Red Bull energy drinks per day, and a handful of dry cereal, going from 231 pounds to 132 pounds.

Saying the expensive Red Bull diet ($20-28 per day) was not a conscious decision at first, the reckless Brooke Robertson said.

"I just started drinking it. I wasn't sleeping, I wasn't eating – I was exhausted. I just continued to drink it because it's an appetite suppressant and I noticed I was losing weight so stuck with it."

Despite the piling up of Red Bull empty cans, Brooke said that she somehow managed to keep her Red Bull energy drink addiction secret from family and friends.

The Red Bull diet sage ended when Brooke Robertson, with her body obviously overwhelmed with the high caffeine and sugar intake, suffered from a heart attack.

"I managed to wean myself off it by being in hospital for that long but I had severe withdrawals – sweating, nausea, shaking. It was an addiction

Discovering a Red Bull energy drink diet might actually kill her; Brooke Robertson now says she maintains her weight through real life conventional exercise and a healthy eating diet.

But the long-term health problems for Brooke persist, she still suffers from heart problems, gets severe pain and cramping in her stomach and bowel, and suffers anxiety attacks from the caffeine and sugar Red Bull addiction, all at the youthful age of 23…but at least she lost weight, right?

# 10

## The Apple Cider Vinegar Diet

Apple Cider Vinegar is a naturally detoxifying product that gently removes toxins from the body, purifies your blood and builds your immune system.

From being almost unknown a few years ago, ACV has gained in popularity to the point that it now forms the basis of many diets and detox plans.

ACV is great for your health - it has antibacterial properties to fight germs, and also balances vitamin deficiencies caused by poor nutrition - but it has wonderful cleansing properties too.

Apple Cider Vinegar is full of antioxidants that neutralize free radicals and help slow down the aging process. It is also great for breaking down mucus in the body and encouraging the lymphatic system to eliminate wastes.

Other Benefits

Here are a few of the other benefits you can expect from Apple Cider Vinegar. Scroll down the page for more details on how to take it.

Increase your energy levels

Apple Cider Vinegar is also excellent to give you a little pep for your exercise regime. Many find increased energy levels and better stamina in the gym... which means burning more calories of course.

Increase your metabolism

Apple Cider Vinegar also has been shown to increase your metabolism. It is thought that this is something to do with its potent combination of vitamins, minerals and trace minerals. Apple Cider Vinegar is especially high in potassium.

Suppress your appetite

Apple Cider Vinegar is a great fat reducing tool. It can be helpful in getting rid of those last few stubborn pounds that a healthy diet and adequate exercise program can't seem to shift. It suppresses your appetite if you get hungry between meals, and discourages you from attacking that second helping.

Reduce bloating

ACV is a powerful diuretic, so it will also ensure you aren't carrying around any unnecessary water weight. Megan Fox spoke recently about her ACV cleanse, "It's just water and raw apple cider vinegar, and it just cleans out your system entirely. It will get rid of, for women who retain water weight, from your menstrual cycle and all that, it gets rid of it really fast."

Stabilize your sugar levels

Apple Cider Vinegar has been shown to stabilize blood sugar levels and reduce insulin spikes after eating. These insulin spikes signal the body to store fat, so you're much better off without them! This is one reason why Apple Cider Vinegar has been touted as a natural supplement for Diabetes sufferers.

How do you take Apple Cider Vinegar?

You have three options for taking ACV as part of your detox. Take it before you eat in water or a fruit juice, add it to your meal as a dressing, or take a bath in it!

Before your meal

Try adding 2-3 teaspoons of ACV in a large glass of water or your favorite juice. It works well with tomato juice.

Be sure to dilute Apple Cider Vinegar as it is highly acidic. Don't drink it straight or you could damage your tooth enamel. Ideally, drink the diluted ACV with a straw to protect your teeth.

If you can't bear the taste or if it feels uncomfortable to drink alternately you can buy capsules from your local health food store.

During your meal

Apple Cider Vinegar can also be used to dress a whole array of foods. Here are a couple of really easy recipes for dressings.

ACV & Olive Oil Dressing
3 Tbsp ACV
3 Tbsp olive oil
Salt, pepper to taste

ACV, Garlic & Canola Oil Dressing
3 Tbsp ACV
3 Tbsp canola oil
1 garlic clove, crushed

Salt, pepper to taste

ACV, Honey & Yogurt Dressing
3 Tbsp. ACV
2 Tbsp. olive oil
1 garlic clove, crushed
3 Tbsp. organic yogurt
1/4 Tsp. honey
Salt, pepper to taste

Mix ingredients well, ideally in something you can really shake up. Add to salads, grilled veggies, fish and chicken, then enjoy!

In your bath

A hot baths with ACV is also a great detoxification method. It is great for flushing out toxins through your skin, and any excess uric acid from the body. Just add 2-4 cups of ACV to a hot bath lie back and soak for 20 minutes!

# 11

## The Grapefruit Diet

Grapefruit diet began in 1930s as the Hollywood Diet. This diet claims that grapefruit contains a special fat-burning enzyme that activated when you eat half a grapefruit along with small amounts of other food for each meal.

At the time, nutrition experts dismissed it as another fad diet, explaining that the 'fat-burning' properties of grapefruit were, in fact, a myth and any weight loss that occurred was due to the extremely low and potentially dangerous calorie intake. With the recent research, grapefruit is back in favor.

A 2004 study led by Dr. Ken Fujioka at the Nutrition and Metabolic Research Center at Scripps Clinic found in a 12-week pilot study that on average, participants who ate half a grapefruit with each meal lost 3.6 pounds , while those who drank a serving of grapefruit juice three times a day lost 3.3 pounds. Additionally, many patients in the study lost more than 10 pounds.

Furthermore, the research indicates a physiological link between grapefruit and insulin, as it relates to weight management. The researchers speculate that the chemical properties of grapefruit reduce insulin levels and encourage weight loss.

The importance of this link lies with the hormone's weight management function. While not its primary function, insulin assists with the regulation of fat metabolism. Therefore, the smaller the insulin spike after a meal, the more efficiently the body processes food for use as energy and the less it's stored as fat in the body. Grapefruit may possess unique chemical properties that reduce insulin levels which promotes weight loss.

The overall study shows grapefruit can play a vital role in overall health and wellness. Whether it's the properties of grapefruit or its ability to satiate appetites, grapefruit appeared to help with weight loss and decreased insulin levels leading to better health.

Eat grapefruit at every meal. Dieter has the choice of eating 1/2 a grapefruit or drinking 8 ounces of unsweetened grapefruit juice and the enzyme is touted to burn away body fat. This diet plan does not allow most complex carbs. Consumption of most vegetables is encouraged and dieters are allowed to prepare them in generous amounts of butter. Consumption of coffee or tea is allowable.

Breakfast Lunch Dinner Bedtime
1/2 grapefruit OR 8 oz. of unsweetened grapefruit juice

2 eggs prepared any way you choose

2 slices of bacon
1/2 grapefruit OR 8 oz. of unsweetened grapefruit juice

Meat any style and any amount.

Salad.
1/2 grapefruit OR 8 oz. of unsweetened grapefruit juice

Meat or Fish any style cooked any way.

Salad

1 cup of coffee or tea.
8oz. glass of tomato juice or 8 oz cup of skim milk.

## The Diet Rules

Drink enough water, a minimum of eight 8-oz glasses/ 64-oz of water every day. Water is essential for all body functions and has no calories.

Follow the exact amount of grapefruit or grapefruit juice suggested. The grapefruit act as a catalyst that starts the "magical" fat burning process.

Although coffee is allowed, dieter should allow themselves maximum 1 cup a day as it affects the insulin balance that hinders the burning process.

Do not eat between meals. Stick to the stipulated meal time.

Dieter should make sure they eat till they are full, so that they won't get hungry later.

You may double or triple portions of meat, salad or vegetables.

Do not eliminate anything from the diet. Especially the bacon at breakfast and the salads. Dieter must eat the bacon and salads. These combinations of food burn the fat, omitting either of the combination will cause the whole thing not to work.

Generous amount of butter is acceptable in food preparation.

Exercise during the diet is not recommended due to the severe restriction of calories. Exercise should only be performed when energy levels are high, and this diet does not provide enough calories for an exercise to be on.

This diet last for 12 days, dieter who decided to continue carry-out the plan must take at least 2 days off before doing so.

# 12

## The Cookie Diet

In 1975, while researching a book on the effect of natural food substances on hunger, South Florida weight loss physician and author Sanford Siegal developed a proprietary mixture of certain amino acids and baked them into a cookie intended to control his patients' hunger. He instructed his patients to consume six cookies (approximately 500 calories) during the day to control hunger, and a dinner of approximately 300 calories in the evening. His "cookie diet" was an immediate commercial success, and within a few years his practice had grown to 14 clinics in Florida and 10 in Latin America. By the mid-1980s, more than 200 other physicians were using Dr. Siegal's approach and products in their own practices. Soon, Dr. Siegal introduced shake mixes and soup with the same hunger-controlling properties.

From 2002 to mid-2006, Dr. Siegal licensed U.S. Medical Care Holdings, LLC to open franchised weight loss centers that used Dr. Siegal's name, weight loss system, and hunger-controlling cookies, shakes and soup. The company opened dozens of centers in the United States and Canada under various names including Siegal Smart for Life Weight Management Centers. The relationship between Dr. Siegal and his former franchisee ended in August 2006. Dr. Siegal no longer supplies his products or licenses his name and weight loss system to USMCH. On September 25, 2008, USMCH filed for Chapter 11 bankruptcy protection.

Three Steps to Success

During the weight-loss phase, with your family doctor's blessing, you'll eat nine Dr. Siegal's Plan 10X variety Dr. Siegal's COOKIE DIET hunger-controlling cookies plus a generous meal. (If desired, one Dr. Siegal's COOKIE DIET brand shake per day may be used to replace two cookies). It's recommended that you have your main meal in the evening but you can have it anytime. The cookies will provide about 500 calories and the dinner 500 to 700. That's a total of 1,000 to 1,200 calories a day. At that level there are no failures; everyone loses weight.

Here are the suggested three steps to reaching your goal weight (subject to your doctor's approval):

Step 1: See Your Doctor

Consult your physician before starting this or any diet. Your doctor may have reasons why you shouldn't begin a diet. Once you begin your diet, check in with your doctor as often as he recommends because people who diet under a doctor's supervision have greater success.

Step 2: Order Cookies

Order a Dr. Siegal's COOKIE DIET Plan 10X 4-Week Starter Kit. Each kit includes a one-month supply of cookies and copies of The Cookie Doctor Cookbook: Countless Combinations of Delicious Meals for Any Calorie-Controlled Lifestyle and Dr. Siegal's Cookie Diet Book.

If you wish, you can also order additional Weekly Boxes of cookies, as well as shakes, dietary supplements, and other products.

Step 3: Lose Weight on Dr. Siegal's Plan 10X™ Eating Plan

The following table shows the Dr. Siegal's Plan 10X Default Eating Plan. This timetable will work for most people who have a typical workday schedule. It assumes that you wake up at around 7am, work from 9pm to 5pm or so, have dinner around 8pm, and go to bed around 11pm. It also assumes that you will have your one "real" meal in the evening (but you can adjust the time to suit your lifestyle). Under this plan, you never go more than two hours without eating in order to reduce the opportunity for serious hunger to develop.

8 AM
2 cookies
(120 calories)

10 AM
1 cookie
(60 calories)

NOON
1 cookie
(60 calories)

2 PM
2 cookies
(120 calories)

4 PM
1 cookie
(60 calories)

6 PM
1 cookie
(60 calories)

8 PM
DINNER
(500-700 calories)

10 PM
1 cookie
(60 calories)


TOTAL DAILY CALORIES:   1,000 to 1,200
TIIME BETWEEN SNACKS: 2 Hours
TARGET WEIGHT LOSS*:    10 to 15 lbs. per Month

# 13

## The Baby Food Diet

Baby Food Diet for Adults?

Overview. The latest fad to hit Hollywood is the Baby Food Diet. Far be it for an actress to need to turn back and try to looking & feel younger (much younger!) or if there is something beneficial to spooning down jars mushy bananas?

The estimation of substituting one, and sometimes two, normal meals a daytime for the tiny fruit and vegetable meals originated from New York style guru Heidi Slimane. The 39-year-old French fashion designer, who has just left Christian Dior to launch his own line, is said to have first coined the phrase 'baby eating' by sticking to baby food for days on end to maintain his slim figure.

As notable in Marie Claire magazine Jennifer Aniston believes the 'purer, nutrient-packed, gluten-free' pots help to keep her trim figure; Reese Witherspoon told a US TV show she's careful to have one adult meal a day. While there is no hardcover of this diet to date, the plan is essentially simple to follow; the dieter eats either all child food or eats one adult meal and baby food for the rest of the day.

Since babies' digestive systems of rules are so young and innocent, most baby food that you'll find at the grocery store is available of added fats, fillers and other additives. It's that simple! No supporting or website has been established as of this writing. The cost of this diet is the price of the baby food.

What we like about this plan. Baby food is available of additives, (Well most of them) pure and full of vitamins. There are many different varieties to select from. Many selections are gluten-free for those on a gluten-free diet. The jars are easy to travel with, and make diet prep work a breeze. Portion control is also a snap. The expense of the Baby Food Diet is low, ranging from $.60 to $1.49. Admit it; it seems so silly, you're thinking about giving it a try.

What we dislike about this plan. No chewing! I think one demand is to be able to chew to feel satisfied. If you are adhering to replace baby food as meal replacements, it is not enough calories a day to keep you full. This diet is so new, there is not much data is on this diet to prove it's worth a try.

How healthy is this plan? It is not. Unfortunately it is just another Hollywood fad dieting. However, if you a replacing that bag of Fritos for a jar of Gerber fruits, it is a positive, healthy modification to your eating habits.

Here's the Bottom Line Swapping baby food for meals will leave you unsatisfied all day long. Sure, you will lose weight but it will be impossible to keep the loss and the project. Using baby food for snack replacement is a healthier option; however, why not use the real plums rather than the pureed style.

# 14

## A Victoria's Secret Models Diet Plan

Your average diet and exercise won't cut it for the annual Victoria's Secret fashion show-the production costs $10 million and approximately eight million people tune in to watch supermodels strut around in panties so all abs and glutes must look perfect. When models say they have good genes and "eat whatever they want" that's only partially true. Victoria's Secret Angel Adriana Lima has opened up about her extreme dieting tricks prior to a major event that we're sure many other top models may adhere too. Take a look at her routine:

•According to the Telegraph, the 30-year-old Brazilian supermodel has been working out with a trainer every day since August. For the last three weeks she's upped her routine to twice a day.

•Lima also sees a nutritionist who measures her muscle mass, fat fashion, and water retention levels. He gives her vitamins and supplements and prescribes protein shakes for energy. And you can forget that eight glasses of water a day rule-Lima drinks an entire gallon to flush out her system.

•For nine days leading up to the November 29 show Lima will consume absolutely no solids. Only a gallon of water a day and protein shakes which include powdered egg.

•Two days before the show Lima will cut out the gallon of water and just drink a normal amount. And 12 hours before the show Lima will put nothing into her body whatsoever. No water, nada. "Sometimes you can lose up to eight pounds just from that," Lima told the Telegraph.

Sophia Neophitou, the British fashion editor who is chief stylist for this year's Victoria's Secret fashion show equates this route to training for a marathon. "Adriana works really hard at it," Neophitou tells the Telegraph. "It's the same as if you were a long-distance runner. They are athletes in this environment - it's harder to be a Victoria's Secret model because no one can just chuck an outfit on you, and hide your lumps and bumps." It's true-when you have eight million pairs of eyes watching you strut down a runway in revealing lingerie you want to look your absolute best and that doesn't happen overnight. But we're amazed these supermodels don't pass out from hunger, exhaustion, or dizziness on the catwalk!

Still, Lima says all the hard work is worth it since Victoria's Secret has practically made her a household name. "The Victoria's Secret show is the highlight of my life," she told the Telegraph. "Becoming an Angel, once I achieved that, it was a dream come true for me. And I know that after all this is done, when I sit down with my daughter one day, we are going to look back and it's going to be very special."

Hmm. There's no denying Lima is a beautiful woman, but we wonder how a daughter would feel about her mother doing extreme diets and posing for the camera in sexy lingerie? And how would having a hot supermodel mom influence a young girl? With 11 years of being a Victoria's Secret Angel on her resume, perhaps Lima will hang up her wings before her baby girl gets teased about her mom being a MILF.

## How You Should Do a Juice Diet for Quick Weight Loss

Basically during a juice diet for quick weight loss, you should have only juice. After my diet, I found out that citrus fruits were not ideal for such a diet, so I suppose that if I were to go on a juice diet again, I would try to have different fruits. I did of course have bananas some times.

A juice diet involves a lot of juicing. So make sure you have a juicer, or one of those mini blenders. Personally I have a mini blender, but I'm sure a juicer would have been more convenient.

You should make the juice periodically, its best if you can make it just before drinking. Organic fruits and vegetables are best, and make sure you only juice those parts that we normally eat, i.e. avoid things like avocado pits, mango and kiwi skins, etc.

Clean your juicer or blender after using it! I know this can get a bit annoying, but you don't want to get a nasty disease while you're on the fast.

Definitely make sure you have a multivitamin and a fish oil tablet every day when you're on the fast. I have them every day anyway, but it's important to be especially vigilant when you're on any kind of fast.

Drink lots of water during the day.

I have also seen recommendations for having one protein shake a day as well, and having done a juice diet, I think it's a great suggestion.

# 15

## Sip and Starve (Juice Diet)

Juice Diet Recipes for Weight Loss

Juice Diet Recipe #1 – The Ginger Zipper
1/2 apple
6 carrots
1″ slice of ginger

Juice Diet Recipe #2 – Super Slim Greens
5 carrots
1 stalk of celery
1 handful of spinach
1 handful of parsley
Optional – mix in a teaspoon of cayenne pepper

Juice Diet Recipe #3 – The V8
1 small tomato
1/2 a small beet
1/4 of a red bell pepper
1/4 of green bell pepper
2 large carrots
2 stalks of celery
1/2 a cucumber
1/2 a small sweet potato
Optional – add in a teaspoon of cinnamon or cayenne
pepper

Source: http://juicerrecipesnow.com/juice-diet-recipes/

Good Morning Sunshine:
- 1 medium grapefruit, halved
- 2 medium apples, cored
- Fresh Italian Parsley, several sprigs
- 1/2 handful of grapes, seedless

Hunger Pain Be Gone:
- 4 medium carrots
- 2 stalks of celery, leaves and all
- 1 handful of parsley
- 4 leaves of baby spinach
- 1 dash of tobasco

Stomach Filler:
- 1 small cucumber, skin and all
- 3 celery stalks, including the leaves
- 1 medium apple, cored
- 2 tablespoons of flavorless protein powder

Smile its Morning Smoothie:
- 2 large oranges, skin removed
- 1 medium grapefruit without the flesh
- 6 strawberries
- 1/2 banana
- 2 tablespoons flavorless protein powder
- 1/4 cup ice

Watermelon Beach Quencher:
- 2 cups watermelon, cubed
- 2 cups honey dew, cubed
- 2 cups cantaloupe, cubed
- 1-inch of fresh ginger, peeled and grated

Strawberry Refresher:
- 1/2 cup strawberries, frozen (not in juice!)
- 1 cup orange juice (fresh squeezed, not concentrate)
- 1/2 lemon, squeezed

Carrot Juice Dream:
- 4 large carrots
- 2 stalks of celery (including leaves)
- 1 medium green apple
- Handful of baby spinach
- Several sprigs of parsley
- Lemon and lime juice to taste

Waist Line Buster:
- 5 carrots
- 1 red apple
- 1 small cucumber
- 1 beet (washed well, peeled and sliced)
- 1 celery stalk
- Ginger optional (for more bite)

Hunger Buster:
- 4 carrots
- 3 sprigs of parsley
- 1 small cucumber
- 2 granny smith apples

Source:
http://diet.lovetoknow.com/wiki/Juice_Recipes_for_Weight_
Loss

Remember, once you've made a few smoothies you will understand what kind of ingredients you like best, and then you can just mix and match to make your own drinks.

# 16

## What Stars are on What Diets?

### Gwyneth Paltrow -- The GOOP Diet

In 2008, Paltrow started her own personal lifestyle Web site called GOOP. The Web site includes diet recommendations, exercise ideas and ways to get yourself moving.

GOOP's tag line is "nourish the inner aspect," and it allows readers to sign up for weekly newsletter that focus on one of the subjects: make, go, get, do, be or see.

After the holidays, Paltrow sent out a GOOP newsletter telling readers how she was going to "lose a few pounds of holiday excess."

"You can detox easily and effectively while you continue to eat," Paltrow wrote, "as long as you are cutting out the foods and other substances that interfere with the detoxification process."

The newsletter then went on to describe a seven-day detox diet that has almost every day starting with a smoothie and ending with a dinner of soup.

"I will be suffering along with you to kick-start my year a bit lighter," Paltrow wrote. "Good luck to us all!"

Lawrence said that he was not a huge fan of multiple liquid meals.

"If possible, I like to see food with fiber being eaten, instead of liquid," Lawrence said. "But honestly, in the end, a healthy diet is not about detoxing, it is about eating unprocessed foods. Eat unprocessed food and you will be OK."

### Kim Cattrall -- The Facelift Diet

Can you erase facial lines and depuff your eyes by eating just fish?

Dr. Nicolas Perricone, creator of the the Perricone Weight Loss Diet, thinks so. And so do Kim Catrall and Julia Roberts, who are two of the many celebrities that have been on the Perricone diet.

Perricone believes a diet high in proteins, which according to him have natural anti-inflammatory properties, can decrease the skin's wrinkling and other signs of aging.

His favorite source of protein is organic, wild salmon. In fact, for the first three days of his 28-day plan, the dieter is supposed to eat a four- to six-ounce filet of salmon at every meal. So those who don't like fish need not apply.

The diet also calls for followers to cut out foods that cause water-retention such as refined sugars and fats.

Lawrence said that on a theoretical level Omega 3 does help with skin.

"Having a healthy intake of Omega 3 does lead to less wrinkling," he said. "What you eat can, of course, affect your skin. For example, carotene-rich foods help prevent sunburn naturally. That said, no study has linked this diet to a significant amount of weight loss."

### Reese Witherspoon -- The Baby Food Diet

Hollywood is always trying to look younger, but now it seems some of them are even eating younger -- a lot younger.

The Baby Food Diet consists of substituting one or two meals a day with a jar of baby food. The other one to two meals a day can be regular "adult meals."

Lawrence thinks that this is one of the better weight loss ideas out there because baby food is just mashed fruits and vegetables.

"It is the least processed of the processed foods," he said.

"I love looking at baby food containers," Lawrence said. "If the flavor is apple berry, you turn the bottle to the other side and the ingredients are just apple, raspberries and blueberries."

"If you want to eat tons of baby food," Lawrence added, "Go for it. It is much healthier than what most people are eating, and the best part is there is not a need for extreme portion control. If you want to eat tons of baby food you are most likely not going to gain weight."

He said that because infant digestive systems are immature, the baby food is fairly free of additives and fillers.

And the best part, lunch can cost as little as 60 cents.

## Kate Winslet -- The Facial Analysis Diet

Just five years before her Oscar win in 2008, Winslet gave birth to a healthy baby boy, but kept the more-than-50 pounds she gained while pregnant.

That is, until she met nutritionist Elizabeth Gibaud, who had a revolutionary way for losing weight -- to look at your face.

"I look for markings, facial color and skin texture," Gibaud told the U.K.'s Daily Mail. "This tells me which minerals are lacking."

For example, according to Gibaud, open pores means there is too much acid in your system and having stress lines means you are lacking mineral salt.

In her book, "The Facial Analysis Diet," Gibraud outlines the six face categories that most people fall into and then lists the foods to eat and the foods to avoid. The book promises that if you modify your diet based on your specific face category, you will see results.

## Kelly Osborne -- The Bar Method

The chubby girl from reality TV's "The Osbournes" is no more.

Kelly Osbourne, 25, was featured on the cover of Us Weekly last month for dropping more than 40 pounds. The starlet, whose parents are Ozzy and Sharon, has been dropping weight since appearing on last season's "Dancing with the Stars." Osbourne said she achieved her new figure by controlling her diet and using a dance-based exercise program called the bar method.

According to the Barmethod.com the routine is a mixture of ballet and Pilates. The workout "creates a uniquely lean, firm, sculpted body" by using "the body-elongating practice of dance conditioning."

Lawrence said that the most important thing is to just get up and move.

"As far as exercise is concerned," Lawrence said, "just walk. Find a way to fit walking into your lifestyle. Remember that you are never going to lose a lot of weight through exercise. You will lose the weight by changing your diet, but exercise is going to keep it off."

Osbourne told Us Weekly that she used to weigh almost 160 pounds and despite being in and out of drug rehab three times, the weight was all that was talked about.

"I took more hell for being fat than I did for being an absolute raging drug addict," Osbourne told Us Weekly. "I will never understand that."

Osbourne also keeps a very positive attitude when it comes to weight loss. She doesn't call her weight-loss plan a diet. Instead, she told Us Weekly, it is "a commitment to a life change."

## Jennifer Aniston -- The Zone Diet

Remember when Aniston appeared on the cover of GQ wearing nothing but a necktie -- at 40?

Even "over the hill," Aniston is still looking fabulous. Recently, Gerard Butler, her co-star in "The Bounty Hunter," said that Aniston "has the best legs in Hollywood."

Aniston credits a mixture of the Zone Diet and regular exercise in the form of cardio and yoga for her figure.

In the GQ article, she said that by sticking to the Zone Diet, with occasional splurges, she keeps her body photo-spread ready.

The Zone Diet, created by Dr. Barry Sears, tells followers to eat a 40:30:30 ratio of carbs, proteins and fats.

Lawrence believes the zone diet is too high in proteins.

"You don't need more than 10 percent of your diet to be proteins," Lawrence said. "Bringing it up to 30 percent is unnecessary. There is also a big difference in plant-based proteins and animal-based proteins. The plant-based proteins like nuts and beans are superior to the animal-based proteins. It has been proven multiple times that cultures with high animal-based protein diets have an increased risk of heart disease."

## Amanda Seyfried -- The Raw Food Diet

In her new movie "Chloe," Amanda Seyfried is looking better than ever. She openly credits the raw food diet for her figure.

The diet consists of eating only unprocessed and uncooked foods. The proponents of this diet believe that when food is cooked, enzymes that aid in digestion are destroyed and the positive nutritional effects of the food can be lessened. The diet includes lots of fruits, veggies and nuts, but it also can include sushi or homemade cheeses and yogurts. If you can hand-make it from raw parts, you can eat it.

Seyfried admitted in the April issue of Esquire magazine that the diet is working to keep her slim. Whether or not she enjoys the diet is another story.

"It's intense. And sort of awful," Seyfriend told Esquire. "Yesterday for lunch? Spinach. Just spinach, spinach and some seeds."

But Seyfried suffers for her art.

"I have to stay in shape because I am an actress," Seyfried told Glamour magazine last month. "It's twisted, but I wouldn't get the roles otherwise."

In Lawrence's opinion, the raw foods diet is the best way to lose weight.

"Raw food is a great diet," Lawrence said. "If you are looking to lose weight, it is good to eat foods that are high in water content like vegetables. The raw food diet purports eating foods that are high in water, low in calories and high in nutrition. The reason we are fat is because we are eating processed foods, so a diet that says only eat unprocessed, natural foods is great."

**Jake Gyllenhaal** has built a hero's body to playing the lead role in the new swords-and-sandals action movie Prince of Persia, the Sands of Time.

Here is his typical daily nutritional plan that packed on muscle whilst keeping him lean.

4.45am Pre-workout snack:- Espresso and banana ( a banana would kick start his metabolism and the caffeine provided an energizing boost)
7am Post-workout breakfast:- Egg white omelet on rye bread (after a hard workout you would need to feed the muscles with protein to help the rebuilding process)
9am Early morning snack:- Protein shake ( calorie and protein dense to help synthesize the muscle repair)

11am Mid-morning snack:- Apple or banana and handful of almonds and raisins (natural sugars and good fats to keep the energy up with plenty of fibre)

1pm Lunch:- Two chicken breasts with a huge salad of avocado, broccoli and other dark green leaves and vegetables (a very lean protein meal with good fats, basic carbohydrates)

3pm Mid-afternoon snack:- Protein shake ( ensuring the muscles have every chance to build)

7pm Dinner:- Steak with steamed veg or grilled chicken with couscous (protein with fats to ensure testosterone levels are high for the next days session)

Jake ate little but often which is the key to building muscle and staying lean.

Notice how most of the food intake was over by 3pm. I would get hungry so choose snacks wisely.

He had lots of salads, vegetables and lean meat to keep his blood sugar levels stable throughout the day.

A good formula for building muscle is to eat around 2g of protein per kilogram of bodyweight, and drink lots of water throughout the day.

**Hugh Jackman's** role as Wolverine made quite an impact on the big screen.

For an over 40 male he makes putting on muscles look all too easy.

He ate protein from natural, unprocessed sources where possible (natural real food is unbeatable for growth).

Ate six small meals a day rather than three large ones (maintain blood sugar levels and keep the metabolism firing).

Drink mainly water (you can not build muscles if you are dehydrated).

Avoid all processed foods, and that includes anything that says "99 per cent fat-free" or similar (processed items simply adds to storing belly fat).

The need for good-quality protein either side of a hard workout is also a priority. Use a supplement if needed like a protein powder. (its easy if you are short on time).

Hugh got plenty of amino acids before training and immediately after, and then he would have a slow-acting protein at night-time, such as cottage cheese (Cottage cheese low fat is a good low calorie protein food to keep you from getting hungry).


**Daniel Craig's** role as James Bond was very impressive and he looked fabulous on the beach scenes.

Daniel's eating philosophy

Ate 3 Meals Per Day and 2 Snacks

His diet was strict but flexible. He didn't eat any refined carbs after 2pm (simple sugars).

He also didn't eat any starchy carbs after 5 pm (potatoes, bread, rice, etc).

He ate pieces of fruit and drank 2 liters of water each day.

It was important that he had a post workout snack after every workout.

Daniel Allowed Himself to Drink Alcohol (that's not surprising for James Bond 007 probably a martini shaken but not stirred).

On Fridays and Saturdays he allowed himself to drink a bit of alcohol. (I prefer straight white spirits like Vodka don't use mixers to reduce sugar or low sugar full strength beer like Kilkenny Irish beer).

This made the diet plan easier to follow, because it was realistic.

## A Typical Day on This Diet

Breakfast: 2 Poached Eggs and 2 pieces of Toast (Protein and fats to starts the day with some carbohydrate make sure its a grain based bread)
Snack: Protein Shake -or- fruits and Nuts (Fruit and Nuts is a better choice than a shake unless you are really short on time)
Lunch: Meat or Fish with small amount of Brown Rice -or- Baked Potato (Good proteins and fats which would really fill you up some carbs to provide energy for the afternoon)
Snack: Protein Shake -or- Yogurt with some Nuts (Live bacteria in Yogurt helps digestion and protects against other harmful bacteria)
Dinner: Meat -or- Fish with some type of Leafy Green Vegetables like Salad, Spinach, or Broccoli.(A very good lean protein meal with basic carbs)
Now I looked at Taylor Lautner's diet as how he got so fit but his approach was entirely different.

He started off with a very defined 6 pack because his body fat was already low at 7% but he didn't have much muscle on his body.

He had to 'beef' up so eating was a full-time job or should I say it was his trainer's job to ensure Taylor was feed.

The basic rule for Taylor was eat every 2 hours, eat as much as he liked as long as it was lean and healthy.

WARNING: Lots of people in the fitness industry talk about eating as many calories as you can. This will make you bulky.

That will help fuel your workouts but reality is will only put on mostly fat.

Its not how much you eat but what you should eat. So you have to be-careful unless you are like Taylor.

Further to this Robert Downey Jr 's workout was the same for Sherlock Holmes and Ironman. However he starved himself for Sherlock Holmes as opposed to feeding himself for Ironman.

I would not normally suggest starving yourself is a good idea, unless it was along the lines of strategic fasting (beginning of every month I fast for 2 days over 3 days and it really helps trigger fat loss, Eat Stop Eat explains this method in detail).

Now the above actor's diet is a guide of what to eat.

If you have no idea of how much to eat here is a simple calculation to determine quantity.

After a while hopefully in 3-4 months you will get a feel for how much you are eating, and will not need to count calories.

Calculating Calorie Intake

Anyhow, this is how to set your daily calorie goal;

Your Goal weight x (workout hours per week + 9.5) = daily number of calories

Example to find daily number of calories:
Say you're 180 pounds and want to add 10 pounds of muscle. Your goal weight, then, is 190. If you plan to work out 3 hours a week, do this: Add 3 + 9.5, and then multiply the sum (12.5) by your goal weight of 190. Result: 2,375. That's your daily calorie goal.

Use this key to figure out how many grams of protein, fat, and carbohydrate you should eat each day.

goal weight = grams of protein

half your goal weight = grams of fat

daily calories – [( protein grams x 4) + ( fat grams x 9)] / 4 = grams of carbs

Example to find how much daily protein, fats and carbs:

For your goal weight of 190, you'll eat 190 grams of protein and 95 grams of fat.

For carbs: Multiply 190 by 4 ( to yield 760), and 95 by 9 (to yield 855). Add them together: 1,615. Now subtract that from your 2,375 daily calories, to yield 760.

Divide that by 4. Result: 190.That's your carb goal, in grams.

Determine how many meals you'll eat each day, and then break down your total allotment into equal portions.

It doesn't matter if you eat three meals a day or six as long as you stay within your calorie guidelines, you will see results.

If you like this idea of natural simple whole foods diets. Here is food guide called Turbulence Training Nutrition Plan which details an eating philosophy the same as these actors. It's simple and uses everyday real foods.

I hope this short listing of the actor's diets help you plan your food regime.

It gives good ideas and reinforces of what steps should be taken to look like these actors.

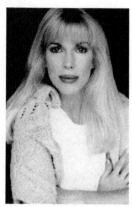

# About the Author

Paige Anders earned her Bachelor's Degree in Creative Writing
and Journalism in the early 90's.   She has published many articles
as a freelance writer for some of the country's most famous
newspapers and magazines.  Her investigative skills have earned
her high praise from her peers and readers. She resides in
Southern California where she lives with her family.

Printed in Great Britain
by Amazon

17894719R00058